What To Expect When Someone Is Dying

By John Antrim

...

For Bill

...

Contents

. . .

The choices we make concerning life and death for loved ones in a situation where they are unable to do so is of most importance. There is no easy way, no set path or map to navigate these difficult circumstances. It is my hope that in reading this guide you will gain an insight and understanding of life support and the end of life which helps you make informed decisions for others, decisions with which you can live peacefully and find solace.

...

1 WHAT TO EXPECT WHEN SOMEONE IS DYING

In 2004 I was working the night shift at a four hundred bed hospital in a suburb of Philadelphia. I was heading down to the emergency room when a middle aged woman entered the elevator. She was sobbing and wiping the tears from her eyes. She looked at me and said, "It's not like when they die on TV, is it?" I took her question as rhetorical and offered no response. She leaned back against the elevator wall, looked towards the light in the ceiling and said, " Dad." Perhaps she was imagining her father might utter some last words or exhale one long final breath. From her appearance the woman looked to have witnessed her father's passing as if she had no

. . .

understanding and perhaps no control over the way in which her father died. *It dawned on me she did not know what to expect simply because no one ever told her what to expect.*

These are the stages of an uncomplicated hospital death.

1) The patient slips into unconsciousness.

2) The patient's heart rate and respirations slow.

3) Skin discoloration may occur at any time during the process.

4) The patient stops breathing.

5) The patient's heart stops beating.

6) A physician declares the patient to be deceased.

To help ensure a peaceful death a steady supply of morphine is administered to the dying patient through a "drip" I.V. A physician determines how much of this strong narcotic is necessary to maintain your loved one in a state of comfort. An overdose of narcotics is not what happens in this situation. The drugs are not used to speed up the onset of death. They are used to keep the patient free of anxiety, pain and fear. The amount of morphine required to do this may vary greatly among different patients.

Sometimes patients continue on respiratory life support (a ventilator) as they depart. In this case the patient appears to be breathing, their chest rising and falling as the ventilator continues to breathe for the patient after they have died. The machine doesn't know the patient has passed and it will continue to perform its duty until it is turned off. After your loved one has passed and is declared deceased by a physician this is "officially" the end.

2   A GOOD DEATH. A BAD DEATH.

There are good deaths, bad deaths and tragic deaths. Tragic deaths may be unexpected or accidental. Young children may be left behind or the death may be of a child. There is no silver lining and there are no true comforts in these situations. There is little or no time to come to terms with the death before it happens. There is no time for saying "Goodbye" or "I love you." No choices are available to determine the circumstances of the dying's last moments. The living are often left confused and overwhelmed by a sudden wave of emotions.

A bad death is one when the patient is suffering emotionally or physically. The patient may be disoriented and / or in pain from their illness.

The idea of a "good death" can be a difficult concept for people of Western societies to understand. In some cultures a good death simply means dying naturally, surrounded by loved ones and leaving no debts behind. A good death may also refer to a death without fear, pain or anxiety. A question to ask yourself is: What would be a good death for you and what would make a good death for others? The following are some criteria contrasting two types of death.

A Good Death

Pain free

Worry free

Treatment following their wishes

Knowing they are loved

Reassurance

Calm atmosphere

Acceptance from family

Loved one(s) present

Guilt free

A Bad Death

In pain

Concern for those around them

Not following their end of life wishes

Confusion

Feeling alone

Noisy, chaotic atmosphere

Family denial of death

Feeling they have left loose ends

Drama

In Chapter 1 I reviewed the stages of an uncomplicated hospital death. In light of discussing an uncomplicated hospital death it should also be noted exactly what having *all* measures taken to sustain life means. There are times when "doing anything it takes" to keep a patient alive is not necessarily the best thing. These efforts can certainly lead to a bad if not a painful death. The following is an account of a lengthy code (aggressive life support measures) of a 92 year old woman, Mrs. L, whom had left her medical decisions up to her daughter. Mrs. L's daughter wanted "everything done" to keep her mother alive.

I was working the night shift at a 650 bed hospital in Nashville. At about 3 AM a Code Blue (cardiopulmonary emergency) was called on the fifth floor. I raced up to the room and found a nurse performing CPR on a 92 year old woman with severe kyphosis (hunchback). The patient's legs were springing up in the air with each compression the nurse gave to her chest. This was due to the patient's deformed spine.

"Her daughter wants everything done," the nurse shouted over her shoulder.

Over the next 50 minutes Mrs. L had:

1) five ribs broken (from chest compressions)

2) multiple bruises on her arms from repeated attempts to gain IV access (older people's veins are tiny and difficult to pierce with a needle)

3) oral and throat lacerations from repeated attempts by the anesthesiologist to place an endotracheal tube in her throat. (her curved spine made this procedure difficult)

After nearly an hour of aggressive CPR, being placed on a ventilator and receiving a large quantity of cardiac drugs, the patient's heart wave returned. She had suffered a massive heart attack. Her brain had suffered damage from lack of oxygen (anoxic encephalopathy). The physician felt another heart attack was imminent and he called Mrs. L's daughter to explain what had occurred with her mother and how he felt a change in code status should be considered. I remember the physician's words verbatim:

"In light of your mother's age and medical state I believe we will only be prolonging her suffering if we continue to treat her aggressively." Shortly after the conversation the doctor told us, "Her daughter wants everything done." We proceeded according to her wishes.

We transported the patient to the Cardiac Catheterization lab where the doctor would attempt to "unclog" her cardiac arteries to prevent another heart attack. He asked me to remain in the lab "just in case they needed a hand." Sure enough, half way through the procedure her heart stopped again. We performed CPR for twenty-five minutes but she was gone. I am sure, that in hindsight, Mrs. L might have reconsidered having "everything done" if she had known what was going to happen to her.

In order for a good death to occur it is important to remember this acronym: **CARES.**

Comfort – the patient should feel no pain or worry.

Acceptance – the living must accept the patient's death so the dying may leave guilt free.

Reassurance – if the patient is assured that everything is alright, he/she will be more at peace.

Emotional support – it is important to meet the needs of the dying.

Saying Goodbye – Goodbyes must be said for the patient to leave peacefully and without worry, guilt or fear.

3 AM I MAKING THE RIGHT DECISION?

Deciding to terminate life support can take a heavy emotional toll. It is usually best for everyone if the decision is made by the patient. Being able to make such a decision indicates the patient has come to terms with his/her death and, as a result, loved ones need not bear the burden of choosing to end life support. With planning, a patient can pre-arrange medical decisions keeping their loved ones from having to make tough choices concerning their medical status. This is known as an "Advance Directive."

An Advance Directive informs the patient's physician what type of treatment the patient wants if they are unable to make medical decisions on their own. Advance directives can describe what levels of care they want to receive depending on how ill they may become, or if they are become unconscious. Advance Directives may also state if a patient wants specific treatments no matter how sick they are. A patient may also state he/she desire Do Not Resuscitate (DNR) status.

A DNR order is a type of Advance Directive which states the patient does not want cardiopulmonary resuscitation (CPR) if their heart stops beating or if they stop breathing. DNR does not mean the patient will not be treated for symptoms which may lead to cardiopulmonary arrest. In healthcare circles it is often said, "DNR does not mean do not treat." It simply states no measures to sustain life will be attempted in the case of cardiopulmonary arrest.

If the choice is left up to you, how do you know you are making the right decision? The right decision must be one you believe reflects the desire of the patient and one you can live with comfortably. To assist you in making an informed decision I offer a questionnaire concerning patient conditions, abilities and Quality of Life which you may find helpful.

Quality of Life *can be measured in the ability of an individual to enjoy life activities.*

4   LIFE SUPPORT QUESTIONNARE (HOW TO REACH A DECISION)

The results of the following questionnaire will give you insight into your loved one's medical state and a prediction of their quality of life after discharge from the hospital.

Score each question from one through five. Give a "5" to represent the healthiest scenario concerning the question and "1" to represent the most unhealthy. The scoring system is based on your judgment of your loved one's medical history, quality of life and current state of being. Take a moment to think before your answer. Quick decisions are not always the best decisions.

Heart: Does your loved one have a complicated cardiac history? Have they ever had a heart attack? Are they currently on life supporting cardiac medicines?   Has their heart been healthy all their life without a problem?

1   2   3   4   5

Cancer: Is your loved one suffering from cancer? If so what stage is the cancer?

1   2   3   4   5

Stroke: At what level are their motor, sensory, vision, language, cognitive abilities and personality affected?

1   2   3   4   5

Lungs: Do they have a history of lung disease? Do they need extra oxygen for life support? Have they ever been told they have COPD?

1   2   3   4   5

Brain: Do they suffer from Alzheimer's disease or dementia? Do they recognize you? Are they able to feed, dress and clean themselves?

1   2   3   4   5

Diabetes: Have they been diagnosed with diabetes?
Do they take insulin daily? Do they have circulatory
problems?

1   2   3   4   5

Kidney: Have they been diagnosed with kidney
disease? Do the need hemodialysis on a regular
basis? Have they ever been told they are "end stage?"

1   2   3   4   5

Blood Pressure: Have they been diagnosed with high
blood pressure? Do they take medication to maintain
normal blood pressure?

1   2   3   4   5

Weight: Are they overweight? Do they have a
"belly?" Have they ever been told they are obese?

1   2   3   4   5

The following questions are scored 3 points for yes, 2
points for undecided and 1 point for no.

Are they able to breathe without the use of a
ventilator?

1   2   3

Are they 78 years of age or younger?

1   2   3

Did they have a good quality of life prior
to admission to the hospital?

1   2   3

After leaving the hospital:

Will they be able to communicate and express their
needs effectively?

1   2   3

Will they be free of pain?

1   2   3

Will they be able to mobilize/get around?

1   2   3

Will they be able to feed themselves?

1   2   3

Will they be able to smile or laugh?

1   2   3

Will they be able to recognize loved ones?

1   2   3

Will they be free of continual life support from this point on?

1   2   3

TOTAL:

_____

What the score means:

50-75

Look at the long term. Life support at this point may be temporary. Speak to the patient's physician, physical, speech, occupational and respiratory therapists to have a better view of the patient's potential for recovery and possibility for a good Quality of Life.

25-50

This score indicates a very challenging recovery for your loved one. Level of future Quality of Life must be examined. Again speak to the physician and therapists to determine the patient's potential for recovery. Removal of life support may be considered.

19-24

A poor prognosis is almost assured. Removal of life support should be a considered. Potential for a good quality of life is nearly absent.

This questionnaire is a tool to help you gain an insight in to the condition of your loved one, their prognosis and the potential for a good quality of life.

The main question is *what would the patient want?*

5   BEING SUPPORTIVE

When one considers how to be supportive at the bedside during the time life support is being withdrawn there must be an understanding of the patient's needs at the end of life. Their main needs are physical and emotional comfort. Prescribed medicines can help with physical discomfort. Emotional support should be given in the manner the patient preferred to receive emotional support when they were able to show appreciation for the effort from others. What made them feel good when they were healthy? Did they need someone physically close by? Did they need their ego stroked? Did they need hugs and kisses or a simple touch on the hand? Did they need to know everything is "alright?" Did they need to know they were loved? Use your knowledge about the patient to help them find peace. A quiet, calm atmosphere is required for the dying to feel it is all right to pass on. I have witnessed deaths where the loved ones of the patient were appropriate, accepting and gracious. I have also been witness to deaths where the next of kin were theatrical, controlling, attempted to be entertaining or cried out at the top of their lungs. Everyone must grieve in their own way but I do not subscribe to the idea that an unruly display of emotion helps the dying experience peaceful conclusion to their life. Until they die, it is about the person in the bed and no one else.

Remember, in order to be most supportive for someone at the end of life you must take care of yourself as well. As I stated earlier, ending life support does not mean the patient will die within

minutes. Sometimes it takes hours, days or weeks.

As a supporter you must hydrate, eat well and get

some sleep. *Take care of yourself.* Whether you are

in the room or not, they are not alone when they pass.

You are still with them through the comfort you

provide in their final surroundings.

6 F.A.Q. – DISCONTINUING LIFE SUPPORT

What is life support?

Life support may be defined as any pharmaceutical, instrumental or therapeutic tool which enables a person to continue living or is used by medical professionals to sustain life. Examples of life support include: mechanical ventilation, hemodialysis, cardiopulmonary resuscitation, defibrillation, pacemaker, feeding tubes and various pharmaceuticals. (These terms are explained in the End of Life Glossary towards the end of this book.) Life support is used to maintain a patient's vital systems while underlying medical problems are treated in hopes of returning the patient to a reasonable quality of life. At times, if a certain level of quality of life is assured, life support may be used indefinitely.

How long does it take a person to die after life support is removed?

The length of time it takes someone to pass after life support is discontinued depends on many factors. Remember, life support is not just a ventilator. Many drugs are considered life support as well.

If a patient has neurological damage and can not take a breath on his/her own the patient will most likely die within minutes when life support, such as a ventilator is removed. Similarly if a drug to keep a patient's blood pressure at a certain level is stopped, it could take any length of time for the patient to pass depending on how sensitive the patient is to the particular drug. If the patient requires hemodialysis to "scrub" their blood and the procedure is stopped death may not occur for days. There is no set time frame. I have taken patients off of ventilators and when they were expected to die within the hour, they lived for days. In other cases I have removed life support and the patient whom our team thought would live for hours passed within minutes.

Are you sure they will die when life support is discontinued?

Considering the poor state of health and the medical needs of the patient when the decision to remove life support is made, death is nearly certain. It is the amount of time the patient will live that is unknown. After removal of life support some patients' lives end in minutes and others last days or weeks. In one case I removed life support from a woman in her mid-fifties who had suffered from childhood tuberculosis. The interior of her lungs were incredibly and irreparably scarred. Breathing was impossible for her without the help of a ventilator. Even with the use of the ventilator it was extremely difficult to fill her lungs with oxygen. Morphine was administered by the nurse and I removed the tubing from her airway an hour later. Her breathing stopped in less than a minute. It was a good death. Her family was present for her end of life. She experienced no suffering. The last words she heard were "We love you," from her sister.

How will I know when they are near the end of life?

If a patient is kept comfortable the end of life will be as simple as absence of breathing and heartbeat. As they approach their moment of death their breathing becomes slow and shallow. Naturally occurring secretions may accumulate in the airway and the patient may develop a "rattle" in their breathing. As long as their rate of respiration is not increasing they are not suffering from this natural occurrence and it may be considered a normal stage of the death process. At times they may take a deep breath approaching a sigh or even a yawn. To put it most simply, they will eventually appear as though they are asleep without breathing. As noted earlier a patient may become discolored at any point during the process of death. Many patients take on a gray pallor as they are about to pass. Others show no discoloration at all.

What can I do to be supportive?

Most people may witness one death, perhaps two during their lifetime. In my opinion many people don't know how to respond but feel as though they should "act a certain way." There is no right or wrong way to act but remember that this is about the patient and no one else. After they have passed it becomes about you and others but while they are in the process of passing on, it is completely about them. So how does one support the dying? First, by being present and remaining calm. Soft voices, "I'm here," "I love you," "Everything is okay." These are things the dying need to hear. Whatever you might consider to be a source of anxiety for a person near death is what you need to leave out of the room. If they liked being touched while they were up and about, one would think this is what they would prefer while lying there. If they weren't the "touchy, feely" type they probably do not appreciate stroking and poking while they await their end. Most often simple hand holding will suffice.

Understanding where the patient is spiritually and emotionally may help guide you in your decisions concerning supportive action for the patient. One may also be supportive of the dying by making informed medical decisions to keep them comfortable and without pain or distress.

How will I know if they are suffering?

Patients undergoing the process of dying are more often than not unable to verbally express their needs or discomforts. This may be due to confusion, exhaustion or the disease process. As with anyone it is possible to recognize the physical symptoms of suffering among the dying. You just need to know what to look for. Facial grimacing, crying out, guarding a certain area or withdrawal of an area of their body from touch, constant shifting or writhing in bed, moaning or groaning, agitation and/or restlessness are all signs of discomfort or suffering. Sedative or analgesic drugs can be of great assistance in helping to alleviate the pain or anxiety a patient may experience during their time of dying.

What medicines do you use to keep the patient comfortable?

Morphine is the drug of choice for end of life comfort. I believe morphine has become the drug of choice for the dying for two reasons. It is among the most powerful pain killers known and it prevents the patient from feeling short of breath and in turn alleviates any suffering caused by inability to breath.

Morphine eliminates "air hunger." It has been reported that morphine will at times interfere with a patient's natural breathing process. If used improperly, this can be true and it is up to the physician to determine the amount of morphine required to provide comfort without suppressing a patient's need to breath. For end of life care, morphine is usually administered as a drip through a patient's intravenous line. I have seen the setting for the drip between 1 milligram/hr to 22 milligram/hr. In neither case was the patient's respiratory drive inhibited. By the time end of life measures are being taken many patients have built up a tolerance to certain drugs and in those cases increased dosage levels may be required for comfort.

Lorazepam (Ativan), diazepam (Valium) and Alprazolam (Xanax) are all members of the benzodiazepine family. They are anti-anxiety drugs used to "slow the brain down" on a conscious level. Again, by the time end of life measures are initiated many patients have built up a tolerance to certain drugs and higher dosage levels may be required to achieve desired effects of comfort.

The drugs mentioned here are by no means the only drugs available for the dying patient's comfort. From my experience they are the most commonly used pharmaceuticals during end of life care.

How will I know when they are gone?

Their breathing will have stopped. Their heartbeat will be absent. More than likely *you will just know.*

7 CONCLUSION

I believe birth and death are the bookends of life. To be present at either should be considered an honor. I have avoided citing religious and personal beliefs in this writing as many different people have various beliefs on the end of life and the implications of removing life support. Some people abide by the school of thought that, "Life support is unnatural. People should be allowed to die in the most natural way possible." If this is their true belief then perhaps pain relief should not be a priority as it is not "naturally" occurring. Others subscribe to the thought, "God gave us these machines to keep the patient alive and they should be used for such purpose." If this is someone's belief then there is little to be said which might change their minds.

Religious beliefs run deep. I am not one to try and

change them though I do suggest reviewing

Ecclesiates 8.8 where it states "No one has the power

over the day of his death." If this is the case then who

are we to initiate life support in the first place? It is

easy to see how different ideas and opinions may

conflict with each other. The end of life is no place

for conflict.

There are those who state "Ending life support

is killing the patient. Ending life support is the

equivalent of murder." Murder is the crime of

intentionally ending someone's life. Discontinuing

life support is far from murder. You are not ending a

person's life. You are letting them pass on to where

they would be without the assistance of technology or

pharmaceuticals. Some people are passionate in their

beliefs and considering the importance of the topic at hand it is understandable.

Decisions in life support should follow the wishes of the patient. If those wishes are unknown one could only hope to provide a peaceful and painless death for their loved one. It is up to loved ones to make decisions which help the patient pass in a way we believe they would desire. When determining if life support is to be discontinued it is important to examine the prognosis of the patient and their potential for a good Quality of Life.

I hope this guide has provided you with a way to organize your thoughts and consider decisions with which you can live and find solace. Thank you.

John Antrim

Contact:

whensomeoneisdying@gmail.com

8 GLOSSARY

Advance Directive: is a set of instructions given by patients specifying what actions should be taken concerning their health if they are unable to make decisions in situations due to illness or incapacity. It appoints a person to make such decisions for them if they are unable.

AICD: (Automatic Implanted Cardiac Defibrillator) an implanted device which monitors the heart's activity. When detecting a life threatening heart pattern it shocks (defibrillates) the heart in hopes of returning it to a normal cardiac rhythm. NOTE: As you may have seen in the movies or on TV when someone is shocked with paddles through their chest in an attempt to save their life the body jerks heavily. The same thing may happen when an AICD is triggered.

Anoxic Encephalopathy: Brain damage due to lack of oxygen. This often happens when a person lapses into a state of apnea (absence of breathing) due to their illness.

Anxiety: a state over activity of the brain creating feelings of uneasiness, worry, dread and fear.

Apnea: the absence of breathing.

Arterial Blood Gas: (ABG) A sample of blood is drawn and tested giving results of the "blood gases" oxygen and carbon dioxide. It may be used as a measure of the current state of the patient's health.

Arrhythmia: an irregular heartbeat.

Assist Control Ventilation: A mode of mechanical ventilation providing full respiratory support to the patient.

Ativan: an anti-anxiety medication.

BiPap: Bi-level Positive Airway Pressure. A device which helps patients breathe more easily without the discomfort of an endotracheal tube in their airway.

Bolus: an amount of a drug administered usually in a large amount to ensure effectiveness.

Brain death: an incurable end of all brain activity.

Cardizem: a drug used to treat heart arrhythmias, high blood pressure and chest pain.

CARES: Comfort, Acceptance, Reassurance, Emotional Support, Saying Goodbye.

CPR: cardio-pulmonary resuscitation.

CVA: Cerebral Vascular Event, more commonly know as a stroke. It is caused by an interruption of blood flow to any part of the brain.

Code: is a term used to issue an to alert hospital staff in the instance of cardiac or respiratory arrest.

Coma: a state of unconsciousness where the patient is unable to respond to the surrounding environment.

Comfort Measures: medical measures to provide pain management and symptom relief.

Decannulation: the removal of a tracheostomy tube.

Defibrillation: a therapeutic shock to the heart to return it to a normal rhythm.

Diagnosis: a statement of what is abnormal about the patient's health status.

DNR: (Do Not Resuscitate) a medical order stating no CPR is to be administered in the case of pulmonary or cardiac arrest.

Dyspnea: an abnormal breathing pattern.

Extubation: the removal of en endotracheal tube from a patient's airway.

Hospice Care: care providing relief of symptoms affecting the patient's health, stress or spirituality.

Hypoxia: an abnormally low level of oxygen in a patient's blood.

Intubation: placement of an endotracheal tube in a patient's airway.

I.V. Drip: intravenous drug administration usually employing a drip chamber to inhibit air bubbles from entering the patient's bloodstream.

Living Will: a type of advance directive

Morphine: a strong analgesic, the drug of choice for end of life care. Helps to suppress the feeling of "air hunger" at end of life. When used properly does not suppress the "need to breathe."

Nonresponsive: a term used to describe a patient who has lapsed into a coma.

Oxygen Level: Room air which we breathe is 21% oxygen. Any percentage of oxygen given above that is considered supplemental. It is administered for the patient's hypoxia in order to maintain a normal blood oxygen level and/or to relieve shortness of breath.

Palliative Care: concentrates on relieving suffering of patients in all stages of disease. Hospice focuses on helping patients at end of life.

Persistent Vegetative State: describes a state in which patients that were in a coma move into a state of arousal but not awareness.

Prognosis: a medical term describing the most likely outcome of an illness

Pressure Support Ventilation: a spontaneous mode of mechanical ventilation helping the patient breathe with less effort than if they were breathing on their own.

Pulse oximeter: a device which provides a measurement of oxygen in the blood.

Telemetry: a medical system enabling health care staff to monitor patient's vital signs remotely.

Terminal Wean: removal of a patient from mechanical ventilation with the expectation of death.

Tracheostomy: a surgical opening in the front/center neck providing access for an artificial airway.

Trach Collar: a "neck mask" placed over a tracheostomy or tracheostomy tube to provide humidified supplemental oxygen.

Quality of life: the ability of an individual to enjoy life activities.

Ventilator: a mechanical device used to move medical gas in and out of the lungs.

Xanax: an anti-anxiety medication

.

Normal Vital Signs

Blood Pressure

90/60 mm/HG – 120/80 mm/Hg

Heart Rate

60-100 beats per minute

Respiratory Rate

12-20 breaths per minute

Remember, what are considered "normal vital signs" differ from patient to patient. The above information may be referred to for reference and is not set in stone. The information is provided as a guideline to help you recognize when the end of the patient's life may be near.

9 RESOURCES

Support Groups:

Elisabeth Kubler-Ross Foundation

"Inspiring Life, Confronting Death"

www.ekrfoundation.org

The Grieving Garden

"A Portable Support Group for Parents Who
Have Lost a Child"

www.thegrievinggarden.com

Center for Loss and Life Transition

"Dedicated to "companioning" grieving people as
they mourn transitions and losses that transform their
lives."

www.centerforloss.com

Grief.com

"Because Love Never Dies"

www.grief.com

Books:

"On Death and Dying"

by

Elisabeth Kubler-Ross

www.ekrfoundation.org

"Closure-The Rush to End Grief and

What it Costs Us"

by

Nancy Berns

www.nancyberns.com

"The Grace in Dying: How We Are Transformed

Spiritually as We Die"

by

Kathleen Dowling Singh

www.kathleendowlingsingh.com

ABOUT THE AUTHOR

John Antrim is a practicing respiratory therapist and educator in southeast Pennsylvania.

Thanks to my wife who has been by my side morning, noon and night since the day we met.

NOTES:

What To Expect When Someone Is Dying

What To Expect When Someone Is Dying

What To Expect When Someone Is Dying
by
John Antrim – 1ˢᵗ edition
ISBN-9781463720315